My Personal Story & Growth Journal

# HAIRLINE
# BLING

## APPLES, EGGS, OILS, & FLARE
### For Scalp, Skin, & Beard

# STEVEN FREE

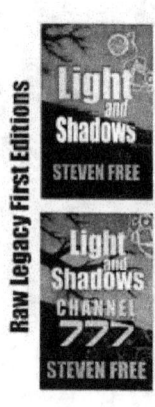
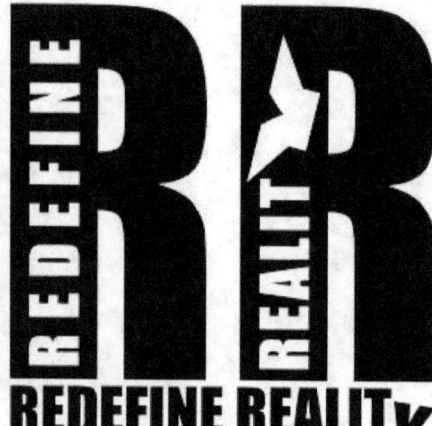
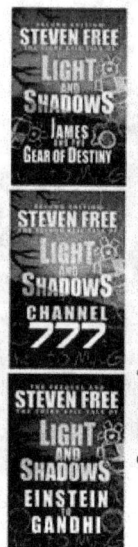

My Personal Story & Journal of Growth

# HAIRLINE

# BLING

## Apples, Eggs, Oils, & Flare
### For Scalp, Skin, & Beard

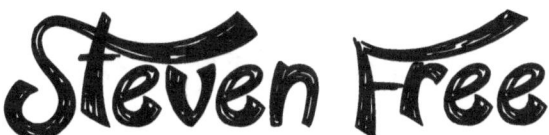

*TO THE MOST HIGH*

## HOW I GREW MY BEARD & SCALP HAIR

# HAIRLINE BLING

## APPLES, EGGS, OILS, & FLARE

## Table of Contents

# Hairline Bling
# Introduction
# By Steven Free

The aim of this book is to chronicle the regrowth of my scalp hair and beard through my personal journal and picture documentation - spanning the course of several weeks into treatment.

When naysayers spoke of myths concerning nutrients which claimed of regrowth, I decided it was ultimately up to me to test natural claims on my own scalp, and publish the photo evidence.

In the beginning, I believed that there was no natural solution to hereditary baldness caused by **DHT**, the "hair killer" hormone, derived from testosterone. That *was* until I discovered how Native Americans and other civilizations used caffeine to combat genetic baldness. Caffeine produces **ATP** within the body and counteracts **DHT** - the "hair killer".

**ATP** rids the body of the possibility of hereditary baldness by the ability to completely shut down **DHT** - the direct cause of the detriment. **ATP** is the body's "*currency*" for the cells. It's the "get out of jail free card" in times of hairline trouble - the unlimited ATM of the cranium.

While **DHT** prevents genetically predisposed cells from receiving nutrients (blocks hair from receiving vitamins and minerals) – the end result is hair fall out due to malnutrition - **ATP** shuts down hereditary baldness by supercharging all of the cells in the body by allowing them to receiving nutrients A.S.A.P. - restoring hair growth to optimal levels for the remainder of the individual's life - well into old age.

I list in detail, the hair treatments and recipes that I apply at least once a day, and let settle for less than one half-hour.

In this book, I document my own transformation - a nightmare that motivated me to form an action plan - and how I came out of that depression into the confirmation of growth.

It is my duty to share my personal story and keep it focused on me throughout. I am a computer teacher by profession and am in no way a certified expert in the field to speak on these issues. However, I am sharing this information in the form of my own personal journey regardless of political correctness, so any information taken herein from this book should be considered as entertainment only.

I cannot call you to action to do what I have done. Please take everything with a grain of salt and listen to your own research and authorities on the issues, if you so choose. Always take the advice of your medical professional before beginning any treatment of any sort.

Take what you read as entertainment because the great Aristotle once said, "It is the mark of an educated mind to be able to entertain a thought without accepting it." Balance this skill within yourselves.

Peace and love,

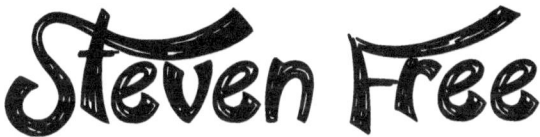

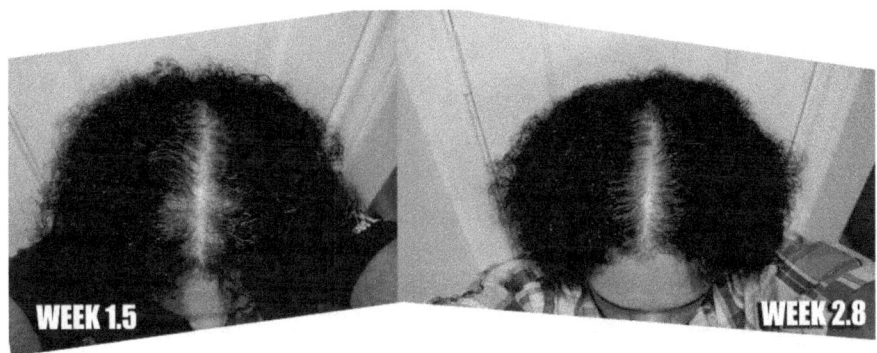

# Hairline Bling
# Chapter 1
# The Dream

Two weeks remained until I was to be in front of the camera to promote my new book, **Light and Shadows: Einstein to Gandhi** - a historical fiction. It was then that I broke the cycle of author-hermitism and looked into the mirror... I mean really looked into the mirror at my appearance after wetting my hair.

I've heard stories and vocal jabs from the likes of comedians in reference to the dilemma and reality of thinning hair.

# "Don't get that hair wet, boy!"

"Don't put any water on it... keep that *thing* dry."

"Because...

"...those hair strands look like six inch gaps when wet!"

Well… I put water on it regardless, and *what do you know*? I knelt down and saw the crown of my head in a new light. Literally a new light.

My previous residence and its dim lighting in the bathroom – hid the problem. While this time, I saw my scalp in a new light within a new residence - as the bathroom was properly lit.

What I saw in the mirror freaked me out. I had known all along that *time* and genetics would eventually catch up with me sooner or later to reap the soul of my hair. I knew that – hereditary conditions and testosterone would lead to an early hair-grave. I felt that balding was inevitable and there was nothing that I could do to stop it – except, to treat my hair somehow through miracle.

As I stared in the mirror - a visualization set. I knew that public swimming was out of the question for me because of the water shrinkage factor to hair – when fully wet. It would be a public embarrassment – I thought. Stringy lifeless clumps - spaced out between one inch gaps – made the bulk of my fear. Being really worried about my image - stress kicked into high gear.

I had a horrid dream that night of losing my confidence. As I awoke, I began to assure myself that my condition wasn't the end of beauty – and that I was just entering a new phase in life.

In response, I began to except that I was not *my hair* and that *my hair* does not change my *character*.

However, a new plan arose from that dream - awakening something that managed the crisis – and lead me to the solution. *See page 63 and 69.

# Hairline Bling
# Chapter 2
# Treat it like a Plant

A hair in the scalp is akin to a plant in the ground. They are both very similar in the needing of nutrients, natural grow aids (fertilizer), and the correct pH balance of their medium (soil or scalp). They both have roots. They both need attention, constantly to thrive and grow.

Both hair and plant need the best ground medium to grow - one which has plenty of circulation for oxygen and minerals to reach the roots.

There are many correlations to waking life also being akin to a something planted. Dreams are grown by constant effort and care – so once manifested – the plant and its blessing will be enjoyed fully - once harvest arrives.

The end result of a dream manifested – is a redefined reality.

Dreams take work. Raising a plant takes work. Hair regrowth is a workout. The same in fact as one would treat their bodies in a gym.

Results are not instant – however – in time – all will be revealed of your faith in action towards your goal.

I remember commercials for the famed *Chia Pet* - an *As-Seen-On-TV* product made that was a clay-like sculpture of an animal. Later the product line included a bust of a person's head - including a seed packet to be spread across its surface and then watered – so that grass would grow to appear as hair on the clay figurine of a person.

Our very scalp is akin to a field where we must nurture, grow, and watch the harvest come to full fruition.

As growers know - a plant or crop needs more nutrients than the actual soil probably provides. These plants need more of what it takes to grow to completion. They require a boost in nutrients that the soil may be missing at the time of potential growth.

Feed your scalp and hair the food it needs and craves to stay alive and thriving. Treat your *soil* which is your *scalp*. And treat your *hair* like a *plant*!

# Hairline Bling

# Chapter 3

# Key Nutes for Hair Growth

**Nutrients** or **nutes** for short, are <u>**vital keys**</u> to the **functioning** of our bodies in order to <u>**survive**</u> and <u>**grow**</u>.

**Nutrients** include both **dietary minerals** and **vitamins**. **Minerals** are substances of a **chemical structure** that can be **found in the ground**, such as **iron** or **copper**, while **vitamins** are **organic** substances **found in foods** that help the body to be healthy.

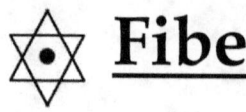 # Fiber

(Found in dark-colored veggies, beans, grains, spaghetti, bran flakes, oats, raspberries, pears, apples, artichoke, broccoli, etc.)

- Adds **durability** to hair follicles
- Facilitates **production** of **melanin**, the **pigment** that gives skin, hair, and eyes their color.
- The average dietary **fiber** intake is around 11 grams. 25-40 grams of fiber can be ideal for healthy functioning

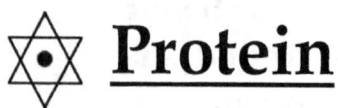 # Protein

(Found in cheese, beans, seeds, lentils, eggs, nuts, meats, fish, etc.)

- Hair is mostly made up of protein
- The main function of protein is to build, strengthen, and repair **keratin**, the fibrous structural protein of hair and nails

# Vitamins:

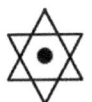 # <u>Choline</u>

(Found in liver, muscle meats, fish – Atlantic cod – salmon, Brussel sprouts, beans, nuts, spinach, peas, wheat germ, eggs, milk, milk chocolate, peanut butter, shrimp, etc.)

- One of the most **powerful nutrients for hair** - considered part of the **B vitamins**
- Supports **construction** of **durable cell membranes** which aid in **hair growth**
- Improves **cell signaling** and **nerve impulse transmission**
- Supports the function of **inositol** which in turn **boosts** the efficiencies of **B complex vitamins**
- Accelerates the **production of Keratin,** the main tissue in hair
- Creates **stronger hair** that **resists breakage**

# 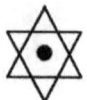 B2 Riboflavin

(Found in beef liver, lamb, milk, yogurt, mushrooms, spinach, almonds, sun-dried tomatoes, etc.)

- **Stimulates cell growth** in hair strands
- **B2 Riboflavin** activates **B6 Pyridoxine** and **B3 Niacin** for **hair growth**

# 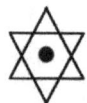 B3 Niacin

(Found in avocado, rice, green peas, Portobello mushrooms, beef, chicken, turkey, liver, tuna, etc.)

- **Improves blood flow** to the **scalp**
- Attracts **oxygen and nutes** from increased **circulation** to the **hair follicle**

#  B5 Pantothenic Acid

(Found in avocado, rice, green peas, Portobello mushrooms, beef, chicken, turkey, liver, tuna, etc.)

- **Key** component in **blood cell** creation
- Essential for **hair growth** and health
- Maintains the transfer of **nourishment** for cells
- Helps **convert** food into **energy**
- Deficiency in **B5** could result in hair loss

#  B6 Pyridoxine

(Found in avocados, bananas, spinach, rice, sunflower seeds, pistachio nuts, prunes, tuna, turkey, chicken, beef liver, etc.)

- Assists with **red blood cell production**
- Studies have shown that a **B6** and **Zinc** combination was able to **stop** the conversion of **Testosterone** to DHT in the skin (**DHT** is the **hair follicle killer** – responsible for patterned **baldness** of the **crown** and **hairline**)

# 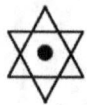 B7 Biotin (A.K.A. Vitamin H)

(Found in eggs, mushrooms, tuna, turkey, avocados, Swiss chard, salmon, sunflower seeds, liver, cheese, cauliflower, whole grain wheat bread, sardines, berries, almonds, bananas, pork, beef, soybeans, etc.)

- **Biotin** is an important component of **enzymes** in the body which assist the **regrowth of lost hair**

# B9 Folate

**Folic acid** is the **synthetic** version of **folate.**
(Found in avocado, asparagus, black eyed peas, lentils, lettuce, spinach, broccoli, mango, oranges, breads, etc.)

- Stimulates hair **growth** by assisting cellular functions
- Deficiency of **B9** could cause hair loss

# 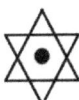 B12 Cobalamin

(Found in beef liver, fish – mackerel – sardines – salmon, fortified cereals, red meat, milk, Swiss cheese, natural yogurt, eggs, shellfish, etc.)

- Assists the formation of **red blood cells**
- Aids **central nervous system** functions

# 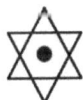 Vitamin A

(Found in cod liver oil, krill oil, carrots, spinach, peaches, bell peppers, winter squashes, sweet potatoes, dark leafy greens, cantaloupe, etc.)

- Produces healthy **sebum**, an oily substance secreted by the scalp, which keeps hair from **drying out** and **breaking off**
- Fights **free radicals** that cause hair to fallout

# 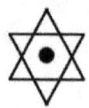 <u>Vitamin C</u>

(Found in oranges, yellow bell peppers, guavas, kale, turnip greens, Swiss chard, spinach, kiwi, broccoli, strawberries, tomatoes, peas, papaya, etc.)

- Helps build **collagen** which is **critical** for growth in **hair strands**
- **B2 Riboflavin** activates **B6 Pyridoxine** and **B3 Niacin** for **hair growth**

# 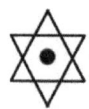 <u>Vitamin D</u>

(Found in fatty fish – catfish – tuna – salmon – mackerel – cod liver oil – sardines, dairy, eggs, beef liver, mollusks, oyster, etc.)

- Maintains normal hair **growth cycle**
- Assists stem cells to enhance and maintain its ability to **produce hair**
- Deficiency can cause **brittle** and **breakable** hair

# 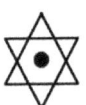 **Vitamin E**

(Found in avocados, sun flower seeds, almonds, spinach, safflower oil, collards, kale, turnip greens, Swiss chard, almonds, shrimp, crayfish, oysters, rainbow trout, wheat germ, olive oil, squash, pumpkin, sweet potatoes, blackberries, mangos, peaches, etc.)

- Stimulates **blood circulation** to the scalp, increasing **oxygen** and **nutrient** passage
- Stimulates **growth** of **capillaries**, increasing the amount of blood sent to the scalp
- Protects hair against **free radicals** which are spread through **pollution** and **smoke** (**free radicals** cause **early aging** of cells which lead to problems such as **thinning** of the hair, **greying**, and eventual **baldness**

# Minerals:

## 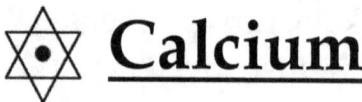 <u>Calcium</u>

(Found in milk, yogurt, cheese, leafy greens, seafood, legumes, sardines, whole grain breads, bran cereals, soybeans, etc.)

- Regulates **cell membranes** critical for **hair growth**
- Deficiency can impact **hair growth**

# 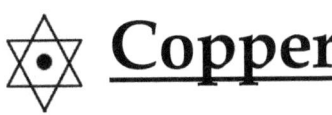 <u>Copper</u>

(Found in avocados, seafood, raw kale, shiitake mushrooms, sesame seeds, nuts, beans, prunes, goat cheese, fermented soy foods -tempeh, miso, fermented tofu, etc.)

- **Copper** and **iron** work together to make **red blood cells**
- **Copper** is a major component of the **outer coating** of **nerve fibers** and **collagen**
- Produces the **antioxidant, Superoxide Dismutase (SOD)**
- **Antimicrobial** properties **fight infection** and **disease causing microorganisms**

# 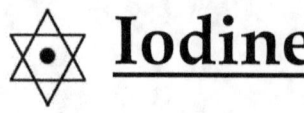 Iodine

(Found in sea veggies – kelp – arame –hiziki – kombu – wakame – seaweed, cranberries, natural yogurt, navy beans, green beans, strawberries, raw natural cheese, potatoes, milk, cod, shrimp, turkey, prunes, tuna, eggs, bananas, corn, lobster, etc.)

- Promotes healthy hair and new growth through its effects on **thyroid function**

# 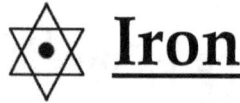 Iron

(Found in red meat, pork, poultry, seafood, beans, dark green leafy vegetables - spinach, dried fruit – raisins and apricots, iron-fortified cereals, breads, and pastas, peas, etc.)

- Critical to **restoring hair growth** as it helps create **red blood cells**
- Deficiency causes **hair loss**

# 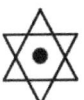 **Magnesium**

(Found in avocados, dark leafy greens – raw spinach, nuts, seeds, fish, beans, whole grains, avocados, yogurt, bananas, dried fruit – figs - prunes, dark chocolate, fish – mackerel – Pollock – turbot – tuna, lentils, whole grain, etc.)

- Aids in **protein infusion**
- Assists in **calcium absorption**
- **Detoxifies the scalp** and **cleanses the skin**
- **Strengthens hair follicles** and **improves longevity** within the hair cycle
- Deficiency can involve **rapid hair loss**

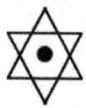 # **Manganese**

(Found in whole grains, nuts, leafy vegetables, tea – black/brewed, seafood, seeds – pumpkin – sesame – flax - sunflower, tofu – firm/raw, etc.)

- Functions alongside of **antioxidants**
- Assists **calcium absorption**
- Essential for proper functioning of **enzymes**
- **Battles free radicals** and **inflammation** by increasing the **superoxide dismutase level**

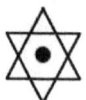 # **Molybdenum**

(Found in beans, nuts, soy, dairy, lentils, peas, etc.)

- Triggers the function of enzymes
- Aids the synthesis of amino acids
- Supports metabolism of compounds

# 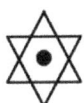 **Phosphorus**

(Found in seeds – pumpkins – squash, chia, sesame, watermelon – flax, cheese – Romano, Parmesan, Goat Cheese, fish – salmon – carp, shellfish – scallops, clams, shrimp, mussels and crab, nuts, pork, lean beef, beans, lentils, etc.)

- **Improves** the condition of **cell membranes**

# 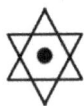 **Potassium** 19**K**

(Found in white beans, greens, potatoes, bananas, clams, yogurt, avocados, salmon, acorn squash, apricots, etc.)

- Assures the **absorption** of vital nutes required for healthy hair
- A potassium deficiency called **Hypokalema** can cause hair to fall out

# 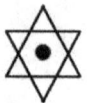 **<u>Selenium</u>**

(Found in nuts – brazil – cashews, seafood – oysters – mussels – octopus – lobster – clams – squid – shrimp, fish – tuna – rockfish – swordfish – halibut – tilapia – mackerel – snapper, whole wheat bread, oat bran bagel, pita bread, English muffin, seeds – sunflower – chia – sesame – flax, pork, beef, lamb, chicken, turkey, mushrooms, whole grains, etc.)

- Supports enzymes, which are proteins that help accelerate chemical reactions
- Accelerates hair growth by assisting proper functioning of hormones and reduces dandruff, as it is utilized in many anti-dandruff shampoos
- Used to treat gray hair
- Anti-flammatory
- Combined with Vitamin E can cure chronic psoriasis and eczema

# 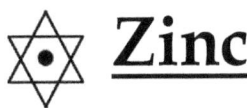 Zinc

(Found in seafood – oysters – lobster - crab, beef, lamb, wheat germ, spinach, seeds – pumpkin – squash – sunflower – chia – flax – sesame, nuts, cocoa, chocolate, pork, chicken, beans, mushrooms, etc.)

- **Assists DNA** and **RNA production,** which is required for the **normal division** of **hair follicle cells,** leading to healthier **hair growth**
- **Balances hormone levels**
- Certain outlying studies show that **aged grey hair returned** to its **original color** when nourished with **zinc**
- may **eliminate dandruff**
- Deficiency may lead to **hair loss**

# Hairline Bling
# Chapter 4
# It's a Workout in Hair.

Are there instant results? Think about efforts put forth in the gym - How a person builds muscle or loses weight through his or her dedication to change. It is a gradual effort - expended over a certain amount of time which sees the results eventually.

Effort and patience – sees results manifest physically.

Attack your dreams with a spirit of optimism along with a determined work ethic and nothing will be able to stop you in the end.

Getting the scalp and hair to optimal health is the same progression as one who applies themselves in a gym.

Know that there is no instant results – only gradually appearances of success until the full culmination of your total efforts.

It's a workout. The vitamins and minerals applied on a daily basis are your proverbial barbell and elliptical. Train with them daily to see success.

Keep the fight and keep pressing on until you achieve your desired results. Never give in to the naysayer - for they produce nothing in the end – only barrenness - the baldness of their field of dreams never brought to reality.

Keep up the efforts for self-improvement.

Be the hard working dreamer that will manifest into reality.

Redefine reality for a better you.

# Hairline Bling
# Chapter 5
# Apples:
# The cleanser.

Apple cider vinegar is primarily used as a rinse for hair. It unclogs gunky build-up of dirt and grime – balanced the pH – and clears the path for new follicles to emerge.

As a natural conditioner, it treats dry - itchy scalp - leaving hair soft, smooth, and shiny.

Its ability to be an anti-tangle mechanism - creates hair that is more easily combed through without snags or breakage.

In addition to conditioning – Apple cider vinegar plays the role of being the most powerful, natural, anti-biotic on earth - as it kills viruses and infections - fungus, pathogens and bacteria (anti-microbial) – and is a cleanser it has the ability to remove buildup that previously blocks the way for new hair to emerge.

Apple cider vinegar does this without stripping the hair of its natural beneficial oils.

Acidic in nature - when diluted with water - apple cider vinegar (**ACV**) pH balances the hair - sealing cuticles along the shaft to prevent split ends - naturally reducing frizz.

The acidity of **ACV** increases blood circulation and lymph flow, wherever it is applied – thus, stimulating hair growth by way of the increased oxygen to the source of application.

Made from the fermenting sugars of apples - the active ingredient in vinegar forms an acetic acid.

**In French, the word *vinegar* means *sour wine*.**

Unfiltered – organic - apple cider vinegar, contains a nutritious substance - full of minerals and a mysterious ether called, *the Mother-* containing various enzymes and strands of proteins.

Not being a major source of vitamins - it does however contain trace amounts of beneficial minerals for healthy scalp and body treatments.

A recommended **ACV** would be **Bragg's Organic Raw Unfiltered Apple Cider Vinegar.**

Let's take a look at nutritional benefits of apple cider vinegar (ACV) in detail:

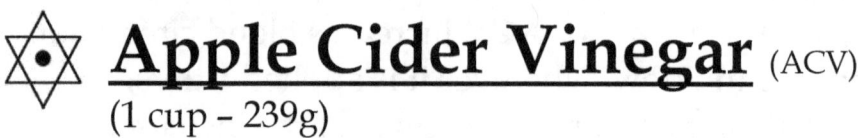

# Apple Cider Vinegar (ACV)
(1 cup – 239g)

## Minerals
- Calcium (16.7mg) *pg. 28*
- Iron (0.5mg) *pg. 29*
- Magnesium (12.0mg) *pg. 29*
- Phosphorus (19.1mg) *pg. 28*
- Potassium (174mg) *pg. 29*
- Zinc (0.1mg) *pg. 29*
- Manganese (0.6mg) *pg. 28*
- Selenium (0.2mcg) *pg. 29*

# Apple Bling Rinse

(Pour thoroughly into hair, soaking the scalp. Allow to set for up to 10 minutes or wash out immediately.)

- Water (8oz.)
- Apple Cider Vinegar (3 table spoons)

# Hairline Bling
# Chapter 6
## Eggs:
## The Muscle

Eggs are one of the best sources of natural protein.

Applying a hair mask using egg yolk will gradually increase the volume of the hair – standing tall for styling – a younger look for confidence – and a fuller - glossier appearance with treatments.

It's the yolk! The all-important supplement to the "muscle" of the strand.

Hair being made-up of proteins (keratin) and amino acids – it is keratin - the fibrous structure of proteins - the visible hair – that is the "muscle".

Amino acids help give protein cells their structure. And eggs are full of proteins, vitamins, and fatty acids that nourish and grow the hair much like muscles within the body.

Making hair stronger to resist breakage and fall out - eggs restore natural oils on the scalp by way of essential vitamins and minerals - with the exception of **Vitamin C.**

Aiding the production of **sebum** (the natural oily secretion under the skin) **Vitamin A** in eggs helps keep the scalp moisturized.

**Fatty acids** within the yolk, **combats dandruff** and **psoriasis** - conditioning the hair into smooth, shining, and manageable texture - while the fatty protein called **Lecithin reduces frizz.**

## Eggs are among the few foods that contain Vitamin D - which maintains a normal hair growth cycle.

Trace amounts of Sulphur within the yolk are known to stimulate the scalp - alongside many of its B-complex vitamins, thought to prevent the premature greying of hair.

## Niacin or vitamin B3 supports energy metabolism in cells - producing new hair growth.

Biotin or B7 renews the roots of strands – for healthy function - making the hair stronger and more durable.

Let's take a look at some of the nutritional benefits of eggs:

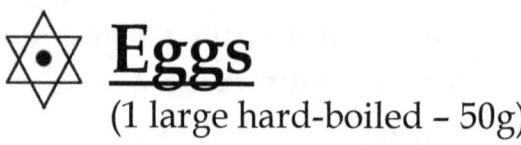 # <u>Eggs</u>
(1 large hard-boiled – 50g)

- Protein (6.29g)

## Vitamins
- **B2** Riboflavin (0.26mg) *pg. 25*
- **B5** Pantothenic Acid (0.70mg) *pg.26*
- **B7** Biotin (8mcg) *pg. 26*
- **B12** Cobalamin (0.55mg) *pg. 27*
- Choline (147mg) *pg. 27*
- Phosphorus (86mg) *pg. 29*
- Vitamin D (43.50IU) *pg. 29*
- Vitamin A (74.5mcg) *pg. 29*

## Minerals
- Iodine (27mcg) *pg. 28*
- Molybdenum (8.5mcg) *pg. 29*
- Selenium (15.4mcg) *pg. 29*

# Hairline Bling
# Chapter 7
## Oils: The Yoga

### Stretching through for Stimulation

Avocado is high in Vitamin E - making it the perfect carrier for caffeine and other nutrients to penetrate scalp and hair.

Avocado oil enhances the absorption of carotenoids (most notably, beta-carotene from Vitamin A. Carotene is responsible for the orange color of carrots and the colors of many other fruits and veggies) and other nutrients.

With the stretching through of scalp penetration and fast absorption – mushed avocado delivered onto the scalp – and allowed to set - has the ability to deliver nutrients directly to the root of the hair.

Yoga or stretching - stimulates the parasympathetic nervous system - which delivers a calming effect - directs our blood toward digestive organs – causing more nutrients to be extracted during digestion.

Certain oils – similar to the benefits of Yoga or Pilates - stimulates blood flow (Vitamin E) in the body and reaches to penetrate the skin with nutrients - delivered straight to the source of need.

### Avocado: The Oily Fruit & Its Ancient Roots

Fossil evidence reveals that avocado trees once existed in pre-Saharan Africa. Specifically originating in West Africa, the species then spread abroad.

Near extinction to its genus – incurred with the gradual drying of Africa, west Asia, and the Mediterranean.

# Ancient Egyptians once used avocado to reduce puffiness under the eyes.

Having knowledge of its restorative properties, it was also applied to the scalp as a **hair mask** for the purposes of conditioning – initiating new growth - and the prevention of hair fall out.

**Once common in Egypt, the Persea genus of which avocado (Persea Americana) faded to near extinction - due to sudden, arid conditions over the region.**

Only Persea Indica remains within the comfortable climate of the **Canary Island Mountains** - located off the southern coast of Morocco.

Avocado oil being high in Vitamin E - makes the perfect carrier for caffeine and other *nutes* (nutrients) to be absorbed directly into the scalp.

Avocado oil – like eggs - enhances the absorption of carotenoids (most notably, beta-carotene from Vitamin A – carotene is responsible for the orange color of carrots and the colors of many other fruits and veggies) and other nutrients.

Let's take a look at more of the nutritional benefits of avocado:

# 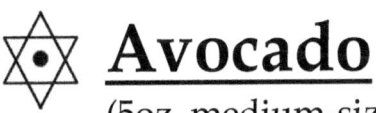 Avocado
(5oz. medium-sized – 150g)

- Potassium (760mg)
- Fiber (10g)
- Protein (3g)

## Vitamins
- **B2** Riboflavin (0.2mg) *pg. 25*
- **B3** Niacin (2.9mg) *pg.25*
- **B5** Pantothenic Acid (2.2mg) *pg.26*
- **B6** Pyridoxine (0.4mg) *pg. 26*
- **B9** Folate (135mcg) *pg. 27*
- Vitamin **A** (220IU) *pg. 27*
- Vitamin **C** (13mg) *pg. 28*
- Vitamin **E** (4.4IU) *pg. 29*

# Minerals

- Calcium (20mg) *pg. 30*
- Copper (0.3mg) *pg. 31*
- Iron (0.9mg) *pg. 32*
- Magnesium (45mg) *pg. 32*
- Manganese (0.2mg) *pg. 33*
- Phosphorus (80mg) *pg. 33*
- Zinc (1.0mg) *pg. 34*

# Hairline Bling

# Chapter 8

# Flare: The Jumper Cables

## Flare: The Stimulation of Caffeine

Caffeine - an organic compound found in several plants and herbs - targets the very thing responsible for genetic baldness – **DHT**.

Having the ability to interact this trace element within testosterone - the hair follicle regains a regulated growth cycle through the stimulation and increased flow of nutrients directly into the scalp by way of topical application.

# Caffeine targets and blocks DHT - the hormone responsible for hereditary baldness.

DHT attaches to hair follicles - preventing the total supply of proteins, vitamins and minerals from nourishing hair – thus causing eventual fall out due to malnutrition.

DHT causes the hair shaft to gradually shrink into non-existence like a plant with no nourishment.

The result? Patterns of baldness like barren grass on an un-kept lawn.

# Caffeine targets DHT by causing root and hair cells to produce a counter response substance called, ATP.

Adenosine triphosphate or ATP for short - is the energy currency of life. A high-energy molecule within every cell of the human body – meant to store and supply cells with needed energy for growth and functionality.

## ATP keeps the hair follicle in an active growth phase by rapidly producing cells within the root.

Caffeine specifically stimulates the cells responsible for hair growth - the **keratinocytes** - epidermal cells which produce **keratin**.

Topical application is the most effective way for caffeine to deliver ATP production into the scalp.

A spray bottle containing caffeine is an effective way to deliver the substance on a daily basis.

## Flare: The Stimulation of Vitamin E

Proper blood circulation is necessary for the scalp to keep hair follicles alive for the receiving of nourishment. Blood circulation is akin to the proper watering of a plant.

Many individuals choose to hand massage the scalp to increase blood flow - however, it is my belief that this method may prove to be more counterproductive and damaging – in that it may lead to loosening existing hairs - rubbing away weaker cuticles - thus causing increased fall out.

It would be advisable to use a method of Flare Stimulation for careful prevention of shedding.

Increases the size of capillaries - Vitamin E - when applied topically to the scalp - grows series of fine branching blood vessels which form a network of internal circulation.

Capillaries are the smallest of the body's blood vessels which make up the microcirculation under the skin and scalp.

Capillary growth leads to improved blood and oxygen flow - delivering nourishment in the form of vitamins and minerals directly to the root of the hair.

## Flare: The Stimulation of Gravity

It has been theorized that the gradual pull of gravity over a standing person – causes the capillaries in the scalp to decrease over time.

It is an explanation for thinning hair leading to eventual baldness in theory.

While some, advise the rubbing of the scalp with the hand to stimulate growth – I believe this method may lead to the pulling and loosening of weaker hair strands – leading to fall out.

By simply tilting the body forward into a downward, stretched position for several seconds – the natural pull of gravity would be enough to increase blood flow to the scalp without massage.

As the face fills with a pressure of blood flow - this surely is a sign that circulation is occurring at the top of the scalp.

This method allows weaker strands to receive needed nourishment from blood flow, without being rubbed out by massage. Repeated stretches downward throughout the day should be enough to give healthy dosages of blood flow to the scalp for increase chance of nutrients to reach the follicles.

# Hairline Bling
# Chapter 9
# Week 1- 2

## - Week 1 -

I woke up from the dream feeling miserable and defeated - feeling like all power or drive were taken from me in one night.

Perhaps my confidence was shot after seeing myself in a new light.

An inner feeling came to the forefront: *I am not my hair*. I am more than my physical shell, and what I have to offer the world, comes from within my shell, and my awareness is an internal knowing.

Howbeit, I must do whatever is required to take the utmost care of myself.

This shell is a vehicle to get me from point A to point B. I must keep it in the best working condition as reasonable possible.

I cannot give up!

This is the spirit of what drives me now.

Through past research into my roots - information on the Native American side of my family - I came across the reference that my native ancestors made use of teas and herbs containing caffeine for hair care.

They kept their crown pristine by rubbing a mixture of the natural substance into their hair. Holding onto this knowledge - they stimulated blood vessels within the scalp and strengthened hair follicles.

I needed to return to that study and find out more of what our ancient people used for health - even spanning into other cultures across the planet.

This is not be the eventual ending of my condition - for I am ever ready now to take action and fight against eventual deterioration.

If I do nothing to care for myself, then I will be following the gradual pattern – leading to a worsened state.

If I do take proper action now - I may be able to turn the table and reclaim my confidence through the tried and true methods that seem to have worked for my ancestors – the same instruction lost in translation - simply lost or intentionally blocked over the centuries - or becoming only an unnoticed footnote in history.

Empowered by hope - I reclaim the condition of my shell for newness - training myself for a better condition.

Using eggs in the treatment – a movie come to mind. Flashbacks of the movie, *Rocky* – and his story of training for an upcoming fight is prevalent.

As a part of his workout regimen, while in the kitchen, he broke a raw egg into a cup in order to drink it for a quick access to protein. Yet in my case, I wouldn't be drinking the egg, instead I would be applying it to my scalp - an out of shape and thirsty scalp - ready for the absorption of nutrients.

The job of protein is to repair, build, and grow. Therefore my first measure of action is to brew a highly concentrated cup of coffee and apply it within the egg yolk - creating a delivery system of stimulated protein to my scalp.

As muscles need protein for repair and growth – likewise - hair is no different.

Hair strands are comprised of an outer shell of protein called keratin - and this - like biceps, pectorals or any other muscle within the body - needs the repair and growth that protein offers.

Thinking of times in the winter where I was unfortunate enough to have a dead car battery - I needed a jump or sudden boost in energy to get me started again. This is where caffeine played the part in reviving my dying scalp with certain java brewed jumper cables.

My recipe and hair mask that I apply every night:

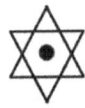 # Rocky Hair Mask Recipe
(Makes a 1-serving treatment)

- 1 large egg
- 3-4 drops of pure Vitamin E oil
- 2-3 broken capsules of cod liver oil
- 1-2 Tablespoons of strong brewed coffee
- 1 drop lavender oil (for optional fragrance)

Brew a strong cup of coffee, then wait for it to cool down to room temperature before adding to the mixture. Excess heat will cook the egg, so be advised to rinse after treatment with cold to lukewarm water only – otherwise – cooked eggs could be logged in the hair.

The mixture of oil and caffeine proves to be an excellent delivery system – absorbed into the scalp when placed topically.

At this point - whether dry or wet - placing hand in my hair meant several strands being removed in one swipe.

Adding a few drops of pure vitamin E oil to the mixture of coffee and egg yolk, for additional Vitamin D - I also used what was available – including snapping the ends of gel caps containing cod liver fish oil - and pouring them into the mix.

This will be my hair mask recipe for week 1 as I look forward to progress in the weeks ahead.

## - Week 2 -

I've never seen this much revitalization before. It reminds me of when I was younger.

When I part my hair now - I get a nice fine parting.

I see fullness coming in - perhaps from the apples (ACV), or eggs – but, my hair has a very different sheen and slickness to it by week 2.

When I comb through my hair with my hands - even when wet – very few hairs pull out – compared to before treatment.

My hair looks and feels stronger, has volume, and stands at attention - whereas in week 1-2 - strands were exhausted and lifeless - appearing limp and dry.

Administering the yolk mixture became less and less messy. Fewer streams of the mixture are left, running down my scalp because of the thickness.

Viewing closely in the mirror, I notice that my roots take to the mixture by clumping together - holding it in place – receiving all of its nutrients head on. (Pun intended)

With my caffeine spray treatments - the coffee applied, now settles along the roots of my hair follicles - preventing drizzle – unlike what occurred in week 1.

Confidence restored – There is hope for restoration. Fewer strands pullout as I maneuver my hand through my hair when completely dry.

It's hard to pinpoint and difficult to word however - I just get a sense that my hair and scalp is much healthier and durable from treatment.

The proverbial out-of-shape scalp and hair of mine has gone through its first phase of a conditioning workout.

I cannot yet grasp, large gains -through immediate visual confirmation as of yet - it is too early to tell – however I'm sure through an inner knowing that my efforts are not in vain because of the fewer and fewer strands that are lodged into my comb and fingers when I brush through.

I see a pattern of hope going into week 3.

# Hairline Bling
# Chapter 10
# Week 3- 4

**- Week 3 -**

Ready for treatment and what do I find? An empty carton. Someone forgot to go grocery shopping - and I was all out of my protein powerhouse at that late hour.

Yet, stumbling across something I did have in the kitchen ready and waiting – something in the kitchen that had ancient roots in hair care – my last avocado.

Creating a hair mask – I let the mixture set in and decided to watch some television. Afterward, it begin to dry.

Washing it out in the shower, I then looked in the mirror to see the shiniest, smoothest hair I had ever witnessed on top of my own crown.

Highly impressed with the avocado mask, the next day I applied the following incredible recipe:

#  Hulk Hair Mask Recipe

(Makes a 2 serving treatment - Refrigerate)

- 1 medium/large avocado
- 1 large egg
- 4-6 drops of pure Vitamin E oil
- 2-3 broken capsules of cod liver oil
- 3-4 Tablespoons of strong brewed coffee
- 1 drop Lavender (for optional fragrance)

Mixing the ingredients thoroughly within a *Ziploc* bag – caused virtually no mess.

A small hole was cut in the corner of the bag and the mixture applied to my scalp like bagged cake frosting.

The natural oils within the avocado played the role of an aggressive conditioner as I surprisingly combed through my hair with ease, even when wet.

The combination of benefits brought by the protein in yolk and nutrients from avocado made my hair much stronger in week 3.

I see slim to no breakage at this point in my treatment. Few if any hairs at all are lodged within my comb after running through with confidence.

Now I can say that I see the light at the end of the tunnel. This would be my first definitive visual proof that the hair treatments are working.

I will be sure to keep this recipe as I move into week 4, as I notice the volume of my hair returning to familiar – younger levels.

Even though new hair growth at this point is hard to determine, I am confident they will emerge soon.

After a week of treatments with the Hulk Hair Mask, I am now able to position and style my hair because of flexible nutrient enriched hair.

I am well pleased with the progress and hope to continue for more amazing results.

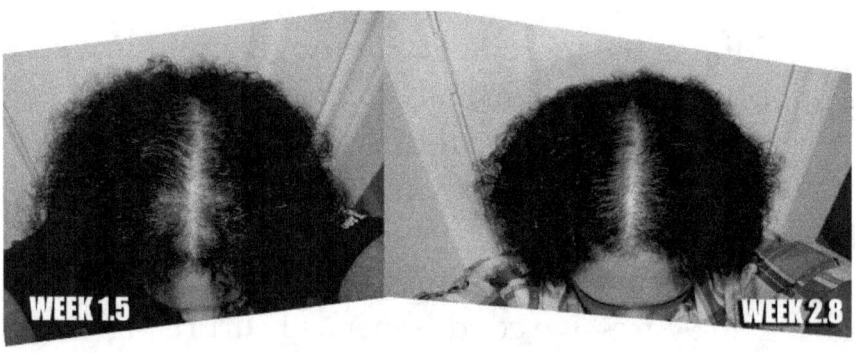

On the last day and a half of week 3, it came to my attention **the effect blueberries have on the hair growth cycle**.

Adding exactly 11 blueberries to the Hulk Hair Mask Recipe, I applied two treatments. The first went well, however I have to mention that the properties in blueberries *can* and *will* dry the scalp fairly quickly.

I will cut back on the amount by adding only two blueberries in the next batch instead of the 11 - or probably end up using them only once a week.

However, leading into week four, I definitely have encountered the brunt of a side-effect of using too many blueberries for hair.

# Hair grows in a 3-stage cycle:

I. **Anagen** Stage (**Growth**)
II. **Catagen** Stage (**Ending** Growth)
III. **Telogen** Stage (**Resting** Phase)

Chemicals found within **blueberries**, called **proanthocyanidins**, stimulate hair growth by moving along the change from **Telogen (resting** stage) to **Anagen** (active **growth** stage) for a longer stay in this position.

## - Week 4 -

Hair texture is changing and appearing thicker. Yet, I have made a grave error – ignoring all warnings of the possible side-effects of using blueberries for hair.

Upon adding exactly 11 blueberries to my Hulk Hair Mask Recipe, I have encountered severe dryness of the scalp due to natural properties within the berry.

All of the natural oil and sheen benefits I had derived from the avocado mixture has seemed to be soaked up by the natural dry-scalp effect that blueberries instill.

My scalp feels extraordinarily dry. The luster and comfort of my scalp is gone and replaced with the itching desert like conditions left by the berry. The hair follicles also seem to be dry. Yet still firm and youthful in appearance - I am led to believe that the blueberry additive actually soaked up all forms and traces of oil in my hair, leaving me with much discomfort of dry scalp.

To remedy this, I am faced with a choice: give up blueberries in the mixture or cut back drastically. I chose the latter.

Cutting down the amount to only one blueberry - I continued to use them in the Hulk Hair Mask Recipe. Instantly I've noticed the positive and beneficial effects of the avocado oil return to my hair.

I have arrived to the conclusion that I should have used only one to two blueberries to the mixture from the beginning and would not advise to continue using them in such a high quantity - or not at all on a consistent basis.

I feel that the berry has done its job by activating the **Anagen stage** or **growth phase** of my hair as a one time basis. Therefore, I may opt to use this method in my recipe one a month instead of on a daily basis.

Despite the slight setback, I have learned much from the process and wish to use it only as a catalyst to start the new hair growth cycle and not for everyday use.

Throughout week four, I will continue to see the promise of well-conditioned hair.

# Hairline Bling
# Chapter 11
# Week 5- 6

## - Week 5 -

In theory a clean shaven or bald head - given the catalyst for growth - would need 8 weeks of growth to be visibly seen at a length between 0.1 to 0.5 inches.

With that said, I expect to see much new hair growth between week eight and eleven where there was no sign of hair before.

This is a workout and a conditioning of the body just as weight lifters condition bodies in a gym – nourishing muscles with vitamins and nutrients throughout the muscles growth cycle.

There is no shortcut to conditioning muscles within the body – so, likewise there is no shortcut to scalp health and follicle growth.

Time is key - and much encouragement to continue into week six is needed because the best is yet to emerge.

## - Week 6 -

I've fallen into another mishap. It was a silly and lazy mistake, yet, can be fixed with time.

I've used an avocado slightly past its freshness date. Upon opening my last avocado… What did I see? Spotted, black ripening - that we all see from an overly oxidized avocado.

It was time for hair treatment once again, and being down to my last resource - I decided to simply scrape off the bad parts and use the good.

In this case it was mostly bad and only little amounts of so-called good left in the fruit. Applying the remainder of what I could salvage for my hair - I let the mixture set in as usual. After more than one half hour later, I rinsed the mask completely and dried my hair. It was only until the next day when I realized my mistake from using the overly oxidized fruit. I woke up the next day with an itching and sore scalp.

Parting my hair – gazing on my scalp - I saw redness due to my use of the overly ripened avocado.

Clearly spoiled and past its prime – I foolishly used the fruit on my hair – unknowingly introducing bacteria and other compounds onto my scalp to settle.

I knew immediately that my mistake was the non-use of fresh fruit – instead trying to be thrifty – I know from now on that I must use the freshest ingredients for my hair and not to cut corners just because it's convenient.

A few treatments later with fresh ingredients – my scalp was healthy and ready to continue the journey.

From here on out it's the usual good growth and conditioning, I've grown accustomed to - and there's no stopping my progress as long as I stay aware of quality control.

# Hairline Bling
# Chapter 12
# Week 7

## - Week 7 -

I'm noticing a new grain of pattern to my hair that wasn't there before. Hair stands at attention with much flex and bounce - in addition to a patterned filling of new growth.

Upon extremely close inspection - I see evidence of new follicles that have emerged through the surface and are peaking above where they weren't before.

New within week 7 are - quick treatments of applying vitamin E oil - solely around the edges of my hairline - once or twice a day - and allowed set in over time.

The oil eventually absorbs into the skin within a matter of hours and provides added support to my treatments.

I imagine this will be a quick solution for those who cannot apply the full hair mask treatment if they are unable to – such as if on vacation or away from the main ingredients for a long period of time.

It would be wise to keep a bottle of pure food-grade vitamin E oil around in a travel case or bag when needed for quick treatment.

The hairline seems sharper than it was in the beginning and is taking well to the oil. I will be sure to keep this quick application up in addition to full hair mask treatments.

# Hairline Bling
# Chapter 13
# Growth Pattern

The average human is born with an average of 100,000 new hair follicles to start life. As we get older, the average daily shedding for an adult is about 50 to 100 hairs a day - which doesn't seem like much when compared to 100,000 scalp hairs in total.

Hairs follow a predictable pattern of growing, stopping growth, and resting within phase.

## Hairs tend to shed during the resting phase.

Scalp hair grows about six inches per year on average, or about half an inch per month.

Each hair grows in the **Anagen phase** for about 2 to 6 years - then stops in the **Catagen phase** during 2 to 3 weeks - entering the **Telogen phase** for 2 to 4 months.

During which it is gradually shed and falls from the head - being replaced by a new hair follicle to start the cycle all over again.

Over the course of a year, the average person normally sheds 18,250 to 36,500 hair follicles in total.

## The Hair Life Cycle:

1) **Anagen** phase (**2** to **5 years** of **growth**)
2) **Catagen** phase (**2** to **3 weeks** of **stoppage**)
3) **Telogen** phase (**2** to **4 months** of **resting**)

# Hairline Bling
# Chapter 14
# It's a Marathon

From being a track and field coach, I can tell you from experience that life is more like a marathon than a race. It is the persistent, constant effort that wins in the end.

Begin your journey and goals with focus, and steady pacing.

Only then will you be able to slap down distractions, jump over obstacles, and push down barriers – simply because you've anticipated the challenge of your marathon.

It's your race. So run it well.

Watch.

There's a bright future a**head** for all of us.

STEVEN FREE – HAIRLINE BLING

Thank you for reading about my journey!!

Be sure to check out my *Light and Shadows* series beginning with *Einstein to Gandhi – Bando – Bando: Trap House – and James and the Gear of Destiny*.

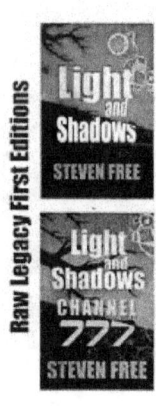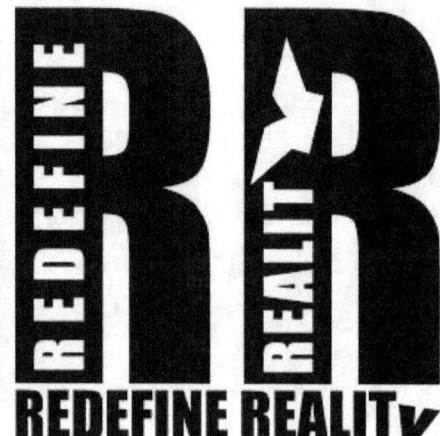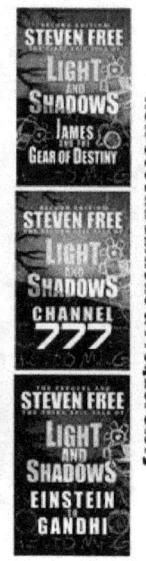

# HAIRLINE

# BLING

Hairline Bling is the cookbook on hair growth – the personal journal of Steven Free and his story of hopeful revitalization. Having gone through a nightmare of confidence and the certain loss of hope – a new plan was formed – a bold action that would soon set in effect the ingredients to glory. A journey laid before him in the form of apples, eggs, oils, and flare – a road leading to the newness of a hairline bling.

# ABOUT THE AUTHOR

# STEVEN
# FREE

---

(Aquarius. Number 11.)

Free's cultural background is Creek Native American, African and German.

Perhaps testing his skill or simply being touched by greatness, Muhammad Ali unleashed a series of playful punching combinations on the back of an unknowing (nearly) 11 year old Free, outside of his class in Michigan.

Free's friend is boxer, TruFE Tru-Iron Mashini.

Free worked as a Production-Assistant for PBS in Washington D.C. while living a short distance away in Queens Chapel, Maryland.

Inspired by his own High School Computer Teacher – years later – following his lead – Free became a teacher of 500+ students in graphic design, multimedia and videogame production in Baltimore, Maryland.

Living in Washington D.C., Free was inspired by French-African cubism painter, JoJo Fekwa – an acrylic painter, who created his own custom DIY custom art frames – made from old flannel shirts that were stretched and stapled over wooden constructs.

Ready.

Paint.

Redefine Reality.

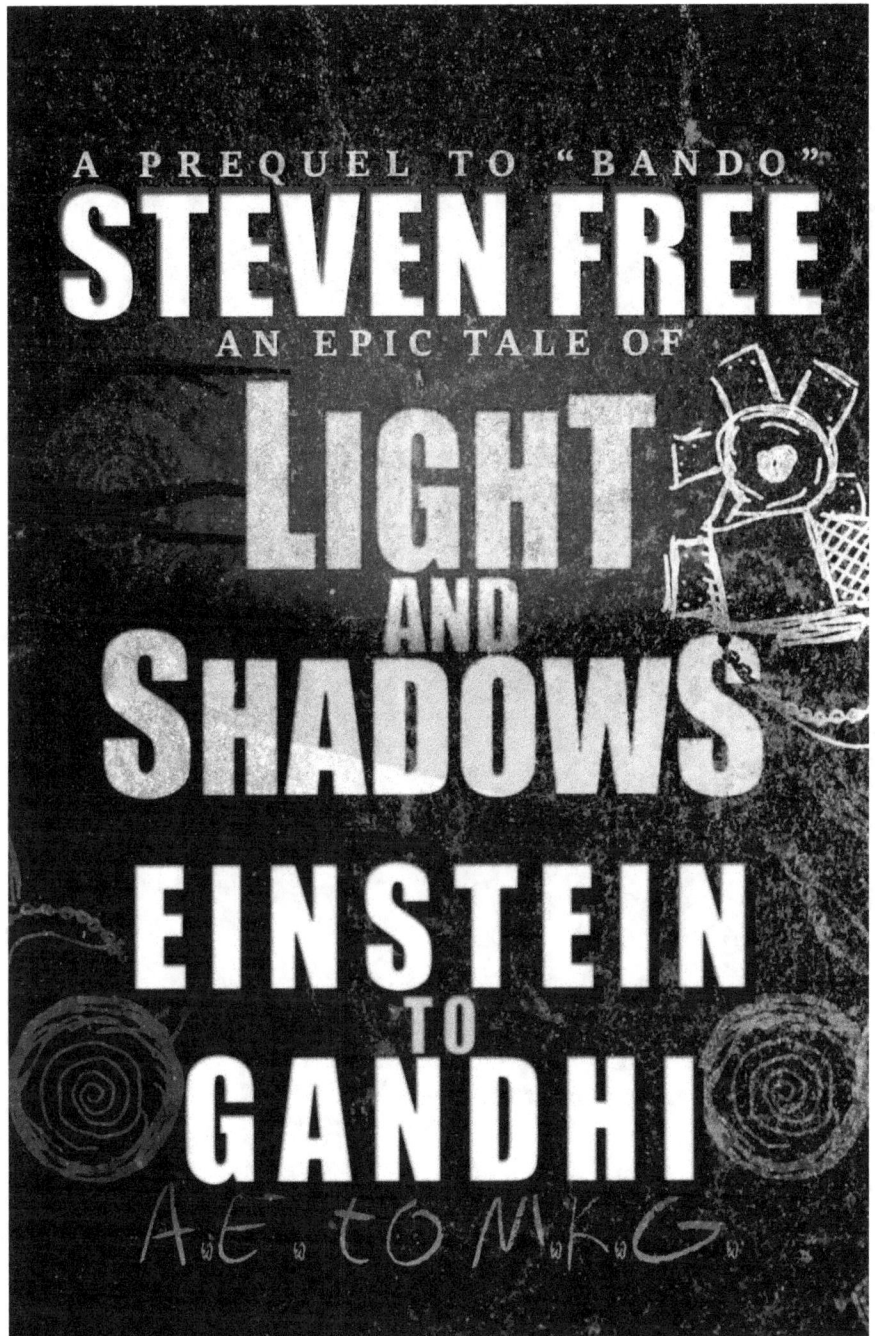

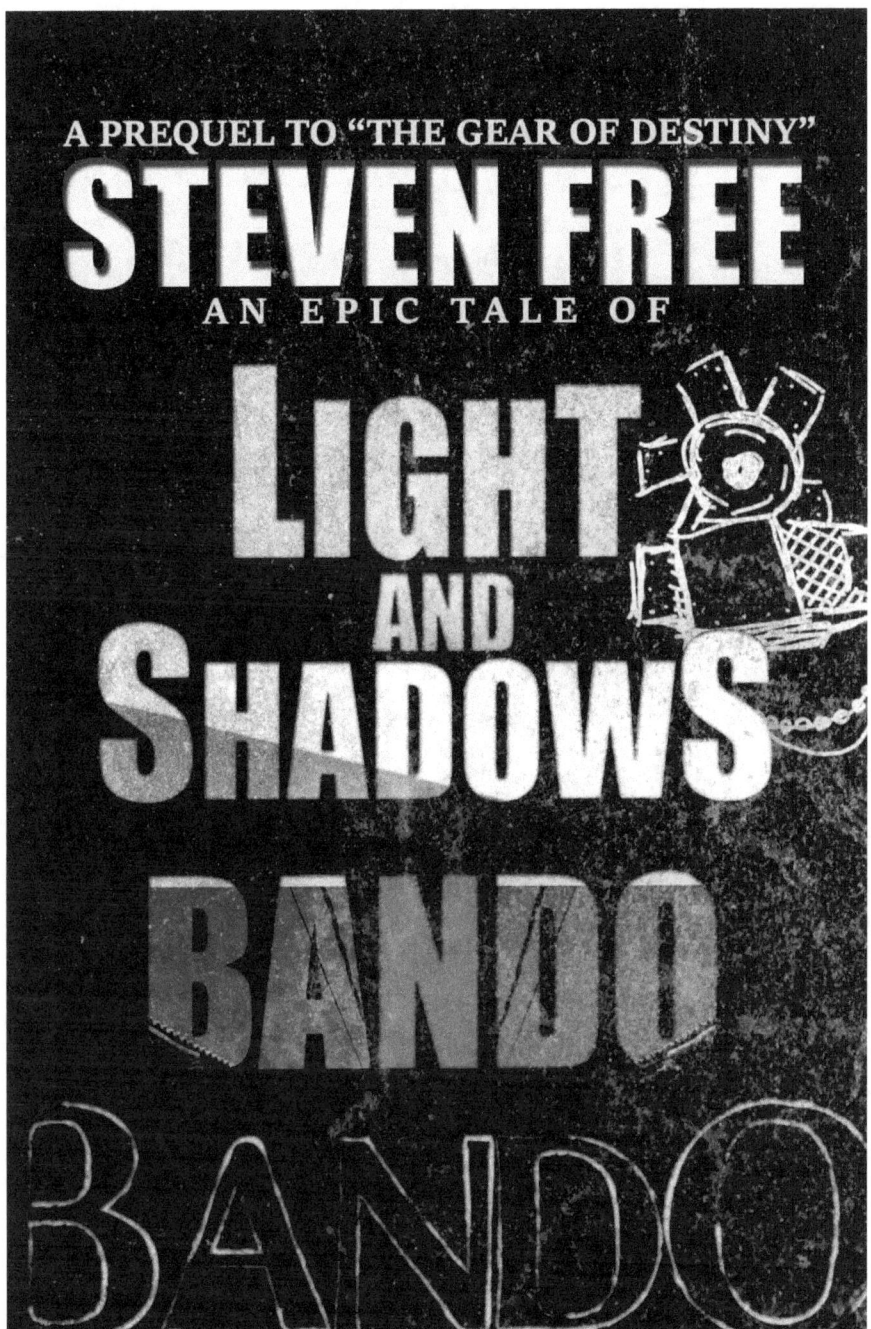

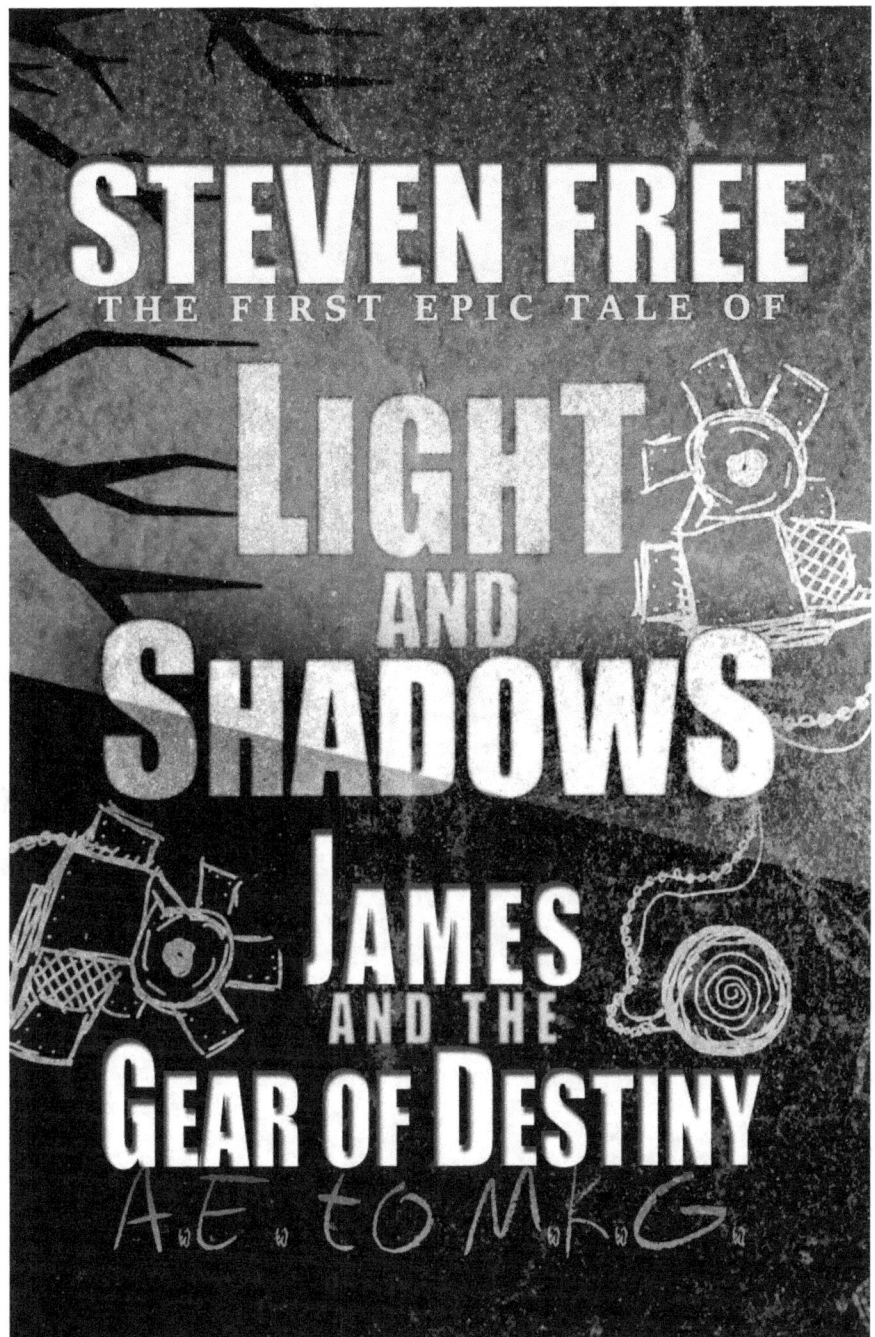